Healing with Essential Oils

Harness Nature's Power for Better Health

Nora Cobbs A.

Table of contents

Table of contents

Introduction

Imagine unlocking the secrets of nature's most potent healing tools, handed down through the centuries, distilled from the essence of plants, flowers, and herbs. From the earliest civilizations to modern wellness movements, essential oils have been a bridge between the earth's natural gifts and human well-being. Their ability to heal, soothe, and transform both body and mind has captured the attention of ancient healers and contemporary wellness experts alike. This book is not just about the therapeutic properties of essential oils—it's about empowering you to reconnect with the natural world and harness its powers for better health.

The history of essential oils traces back thousands of years, where ancient Egyptians, Greeks, and Romans all revered these precious extracts for their medicinal and spiritual properties. The Egyptians, known for their elaborate rituals, were masters of using essential oils in mummification, religious ceremonies, and even personal beauty treatments. Cleopatra herself was said to have used oils like frankincense and myrrh to preserve her youth and enhance her charm. Across the ancient world, essential oils were used in everything from perfumes and ointments to healing balms, symbolizing health, vitality, and divine favor. This rich heritage sets the stage for how these plant-based elixirs have evolved and found a place in our lives today.

Fast forward to modern times, and while we may not be using essential oils in temples or for mummification, their place in contemporary wellness is undeniable. Essential oils are extracted through processes like steam distillation, cold pressing, and resin tapping, preserving the pure essence of plants that are loaded with healing properties. Imagine the complex journey of a single drop of lavender oil—from the flowers grown in fields kissed by the sun, to a precise distillation process that captures its calming fragrance. Or the invigorating rush of peppermint oil, which, through cold pressing, retains its potent ability to refresh and energize. Each bottle holds the concentrated power of nature, ready to be used for therapeutic benefits.

At the core of essential oil use is aromatherapy, a practice that uses scent to promote physical and emotional well-being. Whether it's the soothing scent of lavender to lull you into a restful sleep or the energizing aroma of citrus to wake up your senses, aromatherapy is about more than just pleasant smells. It's the science of how scent interacts with our brain and body chemistry. When you inhale an essential oil, its microscopic particles travel through the olfactory system, directly influencing the limbic system—the part of your brain responsible for emotions and memory. This is why certain scents can calm anxiety, enhance mood, or even improve focus. The benefits of aromatherapy are extensive, offering natural alternatives for stress relief, pain management, and emotional balance.

In today's fast-paced world, where synthetic chemicals often dominate healthcare and wellness products, essential oils offer a return to nature's purity. Their resurgence in modern wellness practices is no accident. People are increasingly seeking natural, holistic solutions to support their physical and mental health.

Essential oils provide an opportunity to move away from harsh chemicals and side effects, opting for remedies that work in harmony with our bodies. The rise of wellness culture has placed essential oils at the forefront, celebrated for their ability to improve sleep, reduce stress, boost immunity, and enhance beauty routines. But essential oils are more than just a trend—they are a testament to the enduring power of nature to heal and sustain us.

As you turn these pages, you will embark on a journey that uncovers the depth and breadth of essential oils, from their ancient roots to their indispensable role in modern life. You will discover how to incorporate these powerful natural remedies into your daily routine, whether it's through diffusing, topical application, or blending your own unique combinations. Each oil carries its own story, and with it, the potential to transform your health, wellness, and emotional well-being.

In the coming chapters, you'll gain an understanding of how essential oils work, the science behind their effectiveness, and how you can use them safely and effectively to address a range of health concerns. This is more than a guide—it's an invitation to experience the beauty, healing, and empowerment that comes from reconnecting with the earth's most precious resources.

As we begin this journey, I invite you to open yourself to the wisdom of nature, rediscover ancient healing traditions, and embrace the potential that lies within these fragrant oils. The next time you hold a bottle of essential oil in your hand, remember the centuries of knowledge and tradition that have culminated in that tiny vial. Let's dive into this timeless practice that continues to evolve, just as we do in our pursuit of health and balance.

This is the beginning of your journey into the fascinating world of essential oils—a journey filled with discovery, healing, and the transformative power of nature. Let's begin.

The Science Behind Essential Oils

When it comes to understanding the power of essential oils, it's important to dive into how these natural wonders actually interact with our bodies. Essential oils aren't just pleasant-smelling liquids—they hold complex chemical compounds that engage our body on a molecular level, producing therapeutic effects that can range from physical healing to emotional balance.

How Essential Oils Interact with the Body

Essential oils are made up of volatile compounds, which means they evaporate quickly and can easily be absorbed by our skin or inhaled through the air. These compounds are tiny enough to penetrate cell membranes, allowing them to be transported through the bloodstream and to interact with various systems within the body. Once absorbed, essential oils can influence the body's nervous system, immune system, and even its hormonal balance. For instance, lavender oil can calm the nervous system, while peppermint oil can stimulate alertness and clarity.

Inhalation is one of the quickest ways for essential oils to enter the body and exert their effects. When essential oils are inhaled, their molecules travel directly to the lungs and are absorbed into the bloodstream, offering almost immediate relief or support, depending on the oil being used. Topical application, on the other hand, allows the oil to penetrate the skin and be absorbed over a longer period of time. When massaged into the skin, essential oils interact with muscles and tissues, providing targeted relief, especially for pain or inflammation.

Chemical Composition and Therapeutic Properties

The healing properties of essential oils come down to their unique chemical compositions. Every essential oil contains a mix of active compounds such as terpenes, phenols, and alcohols, each with its own set of therapeutic effects. For instance, limonene, commonly found in citrus oils like lemon and orange, has uplifting and mood-boosting properties. Linalool, found in lavender, has calming and sedative effects. These compounds work synergistically to provide the therapeutic benefits of the oil.

Beyond aromatherapy, essential oils have antimicrobial, antifungal, and antioxidant properties. Tea tree oil, for example, contains terpinen-4-ol, which is responsible for its strong antibacterial and anti-inflammatory actions, making it popular in skincare for treating acne and other infections. Eucalyptus oil, with its high content of eucalyptol, is known for supporting respiratory health and easing congestion.

By understanding the chemical makeup of each oil, we can better appreciate their diverse healing abilities and how they can be applied in our daily lives. Each essential oil is a complex blend of various natural compounds, and it is this complexity that gives them their therapeutic potency.

The Role of the Olfactory System and Brain Connection

The human brain is uniquely wired to respond to scent, and this connection plays a significant role in the effectiveness of essential oils. When you inhale an essential oil, its molecules interact with the olfactory receptors in your nasal cavity. These receptors send signals directly to the limbic system in the brain, which is responsible for controlling emotions, memories, and even some physical responses like heart rate and stress levels.

Because the limbic system is connected to areas of the brain that regulate mood, hormone production, and the autonomic nervous system, essential oils can directly affect how we feel. For example, inhaling lavender can help reduce anxiety by calming the limbic system, while the invigorating scent of peppermint can stimulate mental clarity and focus. This connection between the olfactory system and the brain explains why certain essential oils are so effective in promoting emotional well-being and stress relief.

Research has shown that essential oils have the ability to influence brain chemistry in profound ways. The scent of an oil can trigger the release of neurotransmitters like serotonin or dopamine, which are responsible for feelings of happiness and relaxation. This is why aromatherapy is such a powerful tool in managing emotions and supporting mental health.

Scientific Studies Supporting the Benefits of Essential Oils

While the use of essential oils dates back centuries, modern scientific research has started to validate their benefits through rigorous studies. Numerous studies have confirmed the ability of essential oils to support both physical and mental health.

For instance, a study published in the *Journal of Alternative and Complementary Medicine* found that lavender essential oil significantly reduced anxiety in patients undergoing surgery. Another study in *Phytotherapy Research* showed that inhaling rosemary essential oil improved cognitive performance and mood in healthy adults, proving its effectiveness in enhancing memory and focus.

Tea tree oil has been widely studied for its antibacterial and antifungal properties. Research in the *Journal of Antimicrobial Chemotherapy* confirmed its ability to kill a variety of harmful bacteria and fungi, making it an effective natural alternative to synthetic antimicrobial agents. Meanwhile, eucalyptus oil has shown promise in treating respiratory issues like bronchitis, as supported by research in the *Journal of Ethnopharmacology*.

These studies not only validate what ancient civilizations already knew, but they also offer a scientific foundation for the continued use of essential oils in modern wellness practices. The growing body of research helps to solidify essential oils' reputation as safe, natural, and effective alternatives for supporting health and well-being.

Getting Started with Essential Oils

Essential Tools and Equipment

When incorporating essential oils into your daily routine, having the right tools and equipment can enhance their effectiveness and make the experience more enjoyable. Here are a few key items every essential oil user should consider:

- **Diffusers**: A diffuser is one of the most popular tools for dispersing essential oils into the air. There are several types, including ultrasonic, nebulizing, and heat diffusers. Ultrasonic diffusers use water and ultrasonic vibrations to release a fine mist of essential oils into the air, while nebulizing diffusers break down the oil into particles without the use of water. Heat diffusers, though less common, use heat to evaporate the oils. Diffusing oils allows for easy inhalation, which is great for improving mood, promoting relaxation, or even purifying the air.

- **Roller Bottles**: These small, portable bottles are perfect for applying essential oils directly to the skin. Roller bottles are typically made of glass and have a rollerball top that allows for smooth, controlled application. They are often used with diluted essential oils, making it convenient to carry your favorite blends for quick, on-the-go use. Whether you're using peppermint for headaches or lavender for stress relief, having a roller bottle in your bag is a great way to ensure you're always ready.

- **Inhalers**: Essential oil inhalers are compact tools that allow you to take a deep, concentrated breath of essential oil when you need it most. These small, tube-shaped inhalers contain a cotton wick soaked in essential oils, making it easy to enjoy their benefits discreetly. Inhalers are ideal for oils that promote mental clarity, focus, or stress relief, like eucalyptus or rosemary.

- **Glass Bottles and Droppers**: For those who like to mix their own essential oil blends, glass bottles and droppers are essential. Since essential oils can degrade plastic over time, it's important to store your oils in dark glass bottles to maintain their potency and protect them from light exposure. Glass droppers make it easier to measure and mix oils with precision.

- **Massage Tools**: If you're using essential oils for topical applications, especially for muscle pain or tension relief, incorporating massage tools like jade rollers, gua sha stones, or massage wands can enhance the experience. These tools help the oils penetrate deeper into the muscles, providing added relief.

Carrier Oils and How to Use Them

Carrier oils are vital when using essential oils, especially for topical applications. Since essential oils are highly concentrated, applying them directly to the skin without dilution can cause irritation or even allergic reactions. Carrier oils help to dilute the essential oil, making it safe for skin contact while still delivering therapeutic benefits.

- **Popular Carrier Oils**: Some of the most commonly used carrier oils include coconut oil, jojoba oil, sweet almond oil, and grapeseed oil. Each has its own unique properties. For instance, coconut oil is highly moisturizing and has antimicrobial properties, making it ideal for skin applications. Jojoba oil closely mimics the skin's natural oils, which makes it perfect for facial applications. Sweet almond oil is lightweight and suitable for most skin types, while grapeseed oil is rich in antioxidants and absorbs quickly.

- **How to Use Carrier Oils**: When using essential oils on the skin, you'll typically mix a few drops of the essential oil with a tablespoon of carrier oil. This not only ensures the essential oil is safely diluted but also helps the skin absorb the oils better. For example, if you're using tea tree oil to treat acne, mixing it with jojoba oil can help moisturize your skin while delivering the antibacterial benefits of the tea tree. Similarly, combining lavender with coconut oil can create a relaxing, soothing body massage oil.

- **Skin Sensitivity**: Different people have varying levels of skin sensitivity, so it's important to do a patch test when using a new oil blend. Apply a small amount of the diluted oil on your inner forearm and wait 24 hours to see if any irritation occurs before applying it more widely.

Dilution Ratios and Safety Guidelines

Diluting essential oils is crucial for safety, especially when using them on the skin. Due to their high potency, using undiluted essential oils can lead to skin burns, irritations, or allergic reactions. Different uses require different dilution ratios, so it's important to know how much essential oil to mix with a carrier oil or base.

- **General Dilution Ratios**: A typical dilution for adults is 2-3% essential oil to carrier oil. This means for every teaspoon (about 5 mL) of carrier oil, you would add 3-5 drops of essential oil. For children, the elderly, or individuals with sensitive skin, it's best to stick to a 1% dilution, which would be around 1 drop of essential oil per teaspoon of carrier oil. If you're making a blend for a massage oil, you might use a lower concentration, around 1-2%.

- **Topical Use**: For direct application on the skin, especially for sensitive areas like the face, it's always better to err on the side of caution. A 1% dilution is usually recommended for facial oils, while a 2-3% dilution can be used for body oils. Essential oils like tea tree or eucalyptus, which have stronger chemical properties, should be diluted more carefully.

- **Aromatic Use**: If you're using essential oils in a diffuser, no dilution with carrier oils is needed. Typically, you'll add 3-5 drops of essential oil to a diffuser filled with water. However, this can vary based on the size of your diffuser and the strength of the oil you're using.

- **Sensitive Populations**: Some essential oils should be avoided by certain populations. Pregnant women, young children, and individuals with certain medical conditions should be cautious when using essential oils. Oils like rosemary and clary sage should be avoided during pregnancy, and eucalyptus or peppermint may not be safe for use on young children. Always research an oil thoroughly or consult with a professional before use.

Best Practices for Storing Essential Oils

Proper storage of essential oils is key to preserving their potency and extending their shelf life. While essential oils don't necessarily "spoil" like food, they can degrade and lose their therapeutic properties over time if exposed to heat, light, or air.

- **Dark Glass Bottles**: Always store essential oils in dark-colored glass bottles, typically amber or cobalt blue. These bottles protect the oils from sunlight, which can break down the compounds and reduce their effectiveness. Clear bottles should be avoided as they offer no protection from light.
- **Cool, Dry Place**: Keep your essential oils in a cool, dry place, away from direct sunlight or heat

sources. The heat can cause the oils to oxidize, which not only diminishes their therapeutic value but can also change their scent profile. A cabinet or drawer is usually a good place for storage. If you live in a hot climate, you may even want to store your oils in the refrigerator to extend their lifespan.

- **Tight Lids**: Oxygen is another factor that can degrade essential oils over time. Always ensure the lids are tightly sealed when you're not using the oils to prevent oxidation. Prolonged exposure to air can cause oils to evaporate or change in chemical composition, making them less effective.

- **Shelf Life**: Different oils have different shelf lives, depending on their chemical composition. Citrus oils, such as lemon or orange, tend to have a shorter shelf life (about 1-2 years) due to their high levels of limonene, which oxidizes quickly. Other oils, like patchouli or sandalwood, can last much longer, sometimes even improving with age. Always check the expiration date or write down the date you opened the oil to keep track of its usability.

By following these guidelines, you can ensure that your essential oils remain as effective as possible for as long as possible, giving you the best results in your wellness journey.

Common Essential Oils and Their Benefits

Lavender Oil

Lavender is one of the most popular and versatile essential oils, known primarily for its calming and soothing properties. It has been used for centuries to help with relaxation and promote restful sleep. Lavender works by calming the nervous system, reducing heart rate and blood pressure, which makes it a go-to solution for stress and anxiety relief. In addition to its calming effects, lavender can also help with minor cuts, burns, and skin irritations due to its antimicrobial and anti-inflammatory properties. For those struggling with insomnia or restlessness, a few drops of lavender oil on the pillow or in a diffuser can significantly improve sleep quality.

Peppermint Oil

Peppermint essential oil is renowned for its refreshing and invigorating properties. It is frequently used to relieve headaches and migraines due to its ability to relax muscles and reduce tension. The menthol in peppermint provides a cooling sensation that can soothe pain and improve circulation, making it a popular choice for treating tension headaches. Additionally, peppermint is known to boost energy levels and enhance mental clarity. Its stimulating aroma helps to wake up the senses, making it ideal for combatting fatigue or enhancing focus during work or study. Whether applied topically (diluted with a carrier oil) or inhaled through a diffuser, peppermint is a powerful tool for both mental and physical rejuvenation.

Tea Tree Oil

Tea tree oil is celebrated for its powerful antibacterial, antifungal, and antiviral properties. It is particularly effective in promoting skin health, making it a popular ingredient in skincare products designed to treat acne, wounds, and infections. The antimicrobial action of tea tree oil helps to kill harmful bacteria and fungi, making it ideal for treating conditions like athlete's foot, dandruff, and fungal nail infections. Additionally, tea tree oil is known to boost the immune system, helping the body to fight off infections and illnesses. It can be diffused to purify the air or applied (properly diluted) directly to the skin for its healing properties.

Lemon Oil

Lemon essential oil is a bright, uplifting oil known for its detoxifying and mood-boosting effects. Extracted from the rind of lemons, this oil is packed with powerful antioxidants, making it an excellent natural cleanser for both the body and the home. Lemon oil supports the lymphatic system, helping to rid the body of toxins and promote healthy circulation. Additionally, its fresh, citrus scent is known to elevate mood and reduce feelings of anxiety and depression. Lemon oil can also be used in skincare for its astringent properties, helping to balance oily skin and clear acne. Inhaling lemon oil through a diffuser is a great way to refresh the mind and create a positive, energized atmosphere.

Eucalyptus Oil

Eucalyptus essential oil is a must-have for supporting respiratory health. Its powerful anti-inflammatory and decongestant properties make it a go-to remedy for colds, coughs, and sinus congestion. Eucalyptus oil works by clearing airways and making breathing easier, which is why it's commonly found in products like chest rubs and steam inhalations. Inhaling eucalyptus oil can help to reduce symptoms of respiratory infections, asthma, and bronchitis. It also has natural antimicrobial properties, making it effective in purifying the air and preventing the spread of airborne pathogens. When used in steam inhalation or a diffuser, eucalyptus oil is excellent for breaking up mucus and clearing nasal passages.

Frankincense

Frankincense is often referred to as the "king of oils" for its powerful healing and spiritual properties. This ancient oil has been used in religious and spiritual rituals for centuries due to its grounding and meditative qualities. Frankincense is known to help calm the mind, deepen breathing, and promote a sense of peace, making it ideal for use during meditation or yoga practice. Beyond its spiritual benefits, frankincense also supports immune function by boosting the body's ability to fight infections. It has anti-inflammatory properties that can help reduce pain and swelling in conditions like arthritis. Frankincense is also beneficial for skin health, helping to reduce the appearance of scars and wrinkles.

Rosemary Oil

Rosemary essential oil is known for its ability to boost memory, focus, and cognitive performance. Its stimulating properties enhance blood flow to the brain, making it a popular oil for improving concentration and mental clarity. Research has shown that inhaling rosemary can significantly improve memory retention and focus, which is why it's commonly used by students or individuals who need to stay mentally sharp. Rosemary is also a powerful hair care oil, known to promote hair growth and reduce dandruff. When massaged into the scalp, it stimulates blood circulation, encouraging healthy hair growth and reducing hair loss.

Chamomile Oil

Chamomile oil, available in both Roman and German varieties, is renowned for its calming effects and ability to reduce inflammation. It is commonly used to alleviate anxiety, stress, and insomnia due to its natural sedative properties. Chamomile also has strong anti-inflammatory effects, making it effective in treating conditions like eczema, psoriasis, and other skin irritations. Inhaled or applied topically (diluted with a carrier oil), chamomile promotes relaxation and can help with sleep disorders. Additionally, it's frequently used in natural skincare for its ability to soothe sensitive skin and reduce redness.

Clary Sage

Clary sage is a powerful oil known for its ability to balance hormones, particularly in women. It is often used to alleviate symptoms associated with PMS, menopause, and other hormonal imbalances. Clary sage works by regulating estrogen levels, helping to reduce menstrual cramps, mood swings, and hot flashes. Its uplifting and calming effects also make it beneficial for emotional support, helping to alleviate anxiety and stress. Clary sage can be diffused or applied topically (with dilution) to provide hormonal and emotional balance throughout the day.

Bergamot Oil

Bergamot essential oil is widely appreciated for its uplifting and mood-boosting properties. Its citrusy, slightly floral scent is known to reduce stress, anxiety, and depression, making it a popular choice for emotional balance. In addition to its mood-enhancing abilities, bergamot is also used in skincare for its astringent properties. It can help to balance oily skin, reduce acne, and minimize the appearance of scars and blemishes. Bergamot oil can be diffused to uplift the atmosphere or applied (diluted) topically for its skin-healing benefits.

Ylang Ylang Oil

Ylang ylang essential oil is prized for its sweet, floral aroma and its ability to reduce stress and promote relaxation. It works by calming the nervous system, making it highly effective for reducing anxiety and promoting emotional well-being. Ylang ylang is also known to support heart health by lowering blood pressure and improving circulation. Additionally, its balancing properties make it a great oil for enhancing mood and relieving emotional tension. When diffused, ylang ylang can create a peaceful, calming environment, and when applied topically (diluted), it can also support skin health.

Cedarwood Oil

Cedarwood essential oil is deeply grounding and calming, often used to improve focus and mental clarity.

Its warm, woody scent has been shown to promote relaxation while enhancing concentration, making it ideal for meditation or work environments. Cedarwood is also beneficial for promoting restful sleep, as it helps to calm the mind and body. In addition, cedarwood is a popular choice for skincare, helping to reduce acne and improve scalp health by balancing oil production.

Ginger Oil

Ginger essential oil is well known for its ability to aid digestion and reduce nausea. It stimulates the digestive system, making it highly effective for treating indigestion, bloating, and stomach cramps. Ginger oil's anti-inflammatory properties also make it a great choice for reducing joint pain and muscle soreness. When applied topically (with a carrier oil), ginger oil can boost circulation and reduce inflammation, making it ideal for those dealing with arthritis or sore muscles.

Geranium Oil

Geranium essential oil is highly valued for its ability to balance hormones and support emotional health. It's often used to regulate the production of sebum, which makes it ideal for both oily and dry skin types. Geranium oil is also known for its skin-regenerating properties, helping to reduce the appearance of scars, stretch marks, and wrinkles. Beyond its skincare benefits, geranium oil is a powerful emotional balancer, helping to alleviate feelings of anxiety and depression. It can be diffused for mood regulation or applied to the skin (diluted) for its beautifying effects.

Patchouli Oil

Patchouli essential oil is often associated with its rich, earthy scent and its grounding properties. Emotionally, patchouli is used to calm the mind, reduce anxiety, and alleviate feelings of stress or nervous tension. Its grounding effect makes it ideal for meditation or relaxation practices. Patchouli also offers significant skin benefits, particularly for dry or aging skin. Its ability to promote cell regeneration helps reduce the appearance of scars, wrinkles, and fine lines. Patchouli oil can be used in skincare routines to soothe inflammation and rejuvenate the skin.

Oregano Oil

Oregano essential oil is a powerful immune booster, known for its strong antibacterial, antiviral, and antifungal properties. It's often used to combat respiratory infections, sore throats, and other illnesses due to its ability to kill harmful pathogens. Oregano oil is highly concentrated and should always be diluted before use, especially when applied to the skin. It can be diffused to purify the air or ingested (with proper guidance) to boost the immune system.

Jasmine Oil

Jasmine essential oil is a luxurious and fragrant oil that has been used for centuries to uplift the spirit and promote confidence. Its intoxicating aroma is known to reduce anxiety, increase feelings of joy, and boost self-esteem. Jasmine is also used in perfumery and skincare due to its soothing properties and ability to promote smooth, radiant skin. It can be diffused to create a romantic or joyful atmosphere or applied topically (with dilution) for skincare benefits.

Cypress Oil

Cypress essential oil is known for its ability to improve circulation and support respiratory health. It is often used to alleviate conditions like varicose veins, muscle cramps, and poor circulation. Cypress oil also has astringent properties, which help to tighten and tone the skin, making it beneficial for reducing the appearance of cellulite. Inhaled through a diffuser, cypress can help with respiratory issues like asthma, bronchitis, or a persistent cough, making it a valuable oil for both skin and respiratory health.

Sandalwood Oil

Sandalwood essential oil is highly regarded for its grounding, meditative properties. It has been used in spiritual and religious ceremonies for centuries due to its ability to calm the mind and promote inner peace. Sandalwood is also a powerful anti-inflammatory oil that can be used to soothe irritated skin, reduce redness, and promote healing. It's often used in skincare for its anti-aging properties, helping to reduce the appearance of fine lines and wrinkles. Sandalwood can be diffused for spiritual practice or applied topically (diluted) for skin care benefits.

Myrrh Oil

Myrrh essential oil is known for its powerful immune-boosting and healing properties. It has been used in traditional medicine for centuries to treat wounds, respiratory infections, and digestive issues. Myrrh's anti-inflammatory and antimicrobial properties make it effective in treating skin conditions like eczema, wounds, and fungal infections. It's also used in meditation and spiritual practices due to its grounding, centering effect. Myrrh oil can be applied topically (with a carrier oil) or diffused to support immune health and emotional balance.

Blending Essential Oils for Maximum Benefit

How to Create Personalized Blends

Creating your own personalized blends of essential oils allows you to tailor the experience to your specific needs, preferences, and health concerns. Whether you're looking to alleviate stress, boost energy, or support sleep, crafting your own blend gives you the flexibility to combine oils that work best for you. When starting out, it's helpful to understand the basic components of a blend and how to balance them to create a harmonious, therapeutic effect.

1. **Start with Your Goal**: Before you begin blending, consider what you want to achieve. Are you aiming for relaxation, pain relief, immune support, or mental clarity? Defining your objective will guide your selection of oils.

2. **Choose Complementary Oils**: Think about oils that complement each other in terms of both

scent and effect. For instance, lavender and chamomile are great for relaxation, while eucalyptus and peppermint work well together for respiratory health.

3. **Experiment with Ratios**: Start with small quantities (1-2 drops of each oil) until you find a balance you enjoy. You can always increase the number of drops, but it's best to start slowly to avoid overpowering the blend.

4. **Test the Blend**: Once you've mixed your oils, test your blend by placing a small amount on your wrist or diffusing it in a room. See how it affects you and if it achieves the desired result.

5. **Keep a Blending Journal**: Track your blends, including the oils and amounts used, so you can replicate successful combinations and tweak those that need improvement.

Balancing Top, Middle, and Base Notes

In the world of essential oils, each oil has a scent profile that can be categorized into three "notes": top, middle, and base. Understanding how these notes work together helps in creating blends that are both balanced and long-lasting.

- **Top Notes**: These are the lightest, most volatile oils, and they are usually the first scent you'll notice when you smell a blend. Top notes are uplifting and fresh but tend to evaporate quickly. Common top notes include citrus oils like lemon, lime, and grapefruit, as well as peppermint and eucalyptus.

- **Middle Notes**: Known as the "heart" of the blend, middle notes provide the main body of the scent. They balance the top and base notes, adding depth to the blend. Middle notes are typically floral or herbal, such as lavender, chamomile, and rosemary. These scents last longer than top notes but not as long as base notes.

- **Base Notes**: Base notes are the foundation of the blend. They are rich, deep, and long-lasting, anchoring the blend and helping to slow the evaporation of the lighter oils. Common base notes include sandalwood, patchouli, frankincense, and myrrh. These oils tend to have a grounding, stabilizing effect on both the scent and the body.

To create a well-balanced blend:

- Start with a ratio of 3:5:2 (3 parts top note, 5 parts middle note, and 2 parts base note). This is a common ratio that provides a harmonious balance.
- Adjust as needed to suit your personal preference. If you prefer a more citrusy, uplifting scent, you may increase the top notes. If you want a more grounding, earthy scent, you might add more base notes.

Suggested Blends for Common Health Issues

Here are some suggested essential oil blends for addressing common health concerns. These blends can be used in a diffuser, roller bottle (with carrier oil), or as part of a massage oil.

- **Stress Relief**:
    - 3 drops Lavender (top note)
    - 2 drops Bergamot (middle note)
    - 1 drop Frankincense (base note)
- This blend is calming, emotionally balancing, and helps to relieve tension and anxiety.
- **Headache Relief**:
    - 2 drops Peppermint (top note)
    - 3 drops Lavender (middle note)
    - 1 drop Eucalyptus (top note)
- The cooling properties of peppermint and eucalyptus work alongside the soothing effects of lavender to alleviate headaches.
- **Immune Support**:
    - 2 drops Tea Tree (top note)
    - 3 drops Lemon (top note)
    - 2 drops Rosemary (middle note)

- This blend has strong antibacterial and antiviral properties, helping to boost the immune system and fight off illness.
- **Sleep Aid**:
  - 4 drops Lavender (middle note)
  - 3 drops Chamomile (middle note)
  - 1 drop Cedarwood (base note)
- The relaxing properties of lavender and chamomile are enhanced by the grounding and calming effects of cedarwood, promoting deep sleep.
- **Respiratory Support**:
  - 3 drops Eucalyptus (top note)
  - 2 drops Peppermint (top note)
  - 2 drops Tea Tree (top note)
- This blend helps to clear airways, reduce congestion, and soothe the respiratory system.

Seasonal and Mood-Boosting Blends

Different seasons and moods call for different essential oil blends. Whether you're aiming to lift your spirits during the cold winter months or celebrate the warmth of summer, essential oils can reflect and enhance the natural energies of the seasons.

- **Spring Refresh**:
    - 3 drops Lemon (top note)
    - 3 drops Peppermint (top note)
    - 2 drops Rosemary (middle note)
- This blend is light, refreshing, and energizing, perfect for the renewal and freshness of spring. It helps clear the mind and invigorate the senses.
- **Summer Sunshine**:
    - 4 drops Orange (top note)
    - 2 drops Bergamot (middle note)
    - 2 drops Ylang Ylang (middle note)
- A bright and uplifting blend, this combination of citrus and floral oils embodies the joy and warmth of summer, boosting mood and energy.
- **Autumn Comfort**:
    - 3 drops Cinnamon (middle note)
    - 2 drops Clove (base note)
    - 3 drops Orange (top note)

- This warm and cozy blend is perfect for fall. The spicy warmth of cinnamon and clove, paired with the bright zest of orange, creates a comforting and grounding effect.
- **Winter Warmth**:
    - 2 drops Frankincense (base note)
    - 3 drops Cedarwood (base note)
    - 3 drops Ginger (middle note)
- A grounding and warming blend, ideal for the colder months. This combination provides emotional comfort and physical warmth, helping to lift spirits during the winter season.
- **Mood Booster**:
    - 4 drops Grapefruit (top note)
    - 2 drops Lemon (top note)
    - 2 drops Bergamot (middle note)
- A bright, citrusy blend that can instantly lift your spirits and boost your energy. This blend is great for diffusing in the morning or during periods of low energy or motivation.

Using Essential Oils for Physical Health

Supporting Immunity with Essential Oils

Essential oils can play a significant role in supporting the immune system by promoting overall health and helping the body fight off infections and illnesses. These oils have powerful antibacterial, antiviral, and antifungal properties that can help bolster the body's natural defenses. When used correctly, essential oils can act as a natural line of defense against harmful pathogens and environmental stressors.

- **Tea Tree Oil**: Known for its potent antimicrobial properties, tea tree oil is one of the best essential oils for boosting the immune system. It helps kill bacteria, viruses, and fungi, making it particularly useful during cold and flu season. Diffusing tea tree oil can purify the air, reducing the spread of germs in your home. Topically, when diluted with a carrier oil, it can be applied to cuts or scrapes to prevent infection.

- **Eucalyptus Oil**: Eucalyptus has strong antiviral and decongestant properties that help protect the respiratory system, one of the body's main lines of defense against illness. It helps clear mucus and open airways, making it easier to breathe during colds or respiratory infections. Adding a few drops of eucalyptus oil to a steam inhalation or diffuser can help to ward off infections and keep the immune system strong.

- **Lemon Oil**: Lemon oil is a powerful antioxidant that supports the immune system by neutralizing free radicals in the body. Its high vitamin C content helps to strengthen the body's natural defenses. Lemon oil also has antimicrobial properties that help cleanse the body and the environment. Diffusing lemon oil or adding it to cleaning products can help eliminate germs and bacteria in your home.

- **Oregano Oil**: Oregano oil is one of the most potent essential oils for boosting immunity, with its strong antibacterial, antiviral, and antifungal properties. It is often used in natural remedies to combat infections and illnesses. Oregano oil can be diffused to purify the air or diluted with a carrier oil and applied to the soles of the feet for immune support. Due to its strength, it should always be diluted properly before use.

- **Frankincense Oil**: Frankincense is known for its ability to support the immune system and reduce inflammation. Its grounding properties help calm the body and mind, which is essential for maintaining a healthy immune response. Frankincense can be diffused or applied topically (with dilution) to support immune health.

Digestive Health and Essential Oils

Essential oils can offer natural relief for a variety of digestive issues, from indigestion and bloating to nausea and stomach cramps. Their ability to stimulate the digestive system and reduce inflammation makes them an effective, natural remedy for promoting gut health.

- **Peppermint Oil**: One of the most widely known essential oils for digestive health, peppermint oil works by relaxing the muscles of the gastrointestinal tract, making it highly effective for relieving indigestion, gas, and bloating. It also helps stimulate bile flow, which aids digestion. Peppermint oil can be applied topically (diluted) to the abdomen or taken internally (with proper guidance) to alleviate digestive discomfort.

- **Ginger Oil**: Known for its anti-inflammatory and stomach-soothing properties, ginger oil is particularly useful for treating nausea, indigestion, and motion sickness. Ginger oil helps stimulate digestion and reduce inflammation in the digestive tract, making it effective for conditions like irritable bowel syndrome (IBS). Diluted ginger oil can be massaged onto the abdomen or inhaled to alleviate nausea.

- **Fennel Oil**: Fennel oil is excellent for supporting digestion, particularly for reducing gas, bloating, and constipation. It stimulates the digestive system, encouraging smooth bowel movements. Fennel oil can be used topically (diluted) in a massage blend for the abdomen or taken internally (with proper guidance) to support digestion.

- **Lemon Oil**: Lemon oil promotes detoxification by stimulating the liver and supporting healthy digestion. It helps to cleanse the digestive system, improve bile production, and reduce indigestion. Adding a few drops of lemon oil to a glass of water (if the oil is food-grade) can help detoxify the body and improve digestion.

- **Cardamom Oil**: Known for its warm, spicy aroma, cardamom oil helps relieve indigestion, nausea, and vomiting. It also has carminative properties, meaning it helps prevent gas formation in the digestive tract. Diffusing cardamom oil or applying it topically (diluted) to the abdomen can support digestive health.

Respiratory Support and Essential Oils

Essential oils can provide powerful respiratory support, helping to clear congestion, ease breathing, and reduce symptoms associated with respiratory conditions like colds, allergies, asthma, and bronchitis. Their anti-inflammatory and decongestant properties make them a natural choice for promoting healthy lung function and respiratory health.

- **Eucalyptus Oil**: Eucalyptus is one of the most effective essential oils for respiratory health, known for its ability to clear congestion and open airways. Its anti-inflammatory and decongestant properties make it an ideal remedy for colds, sinus infections, and respiratory conditions like asthma. Eucalyptus oil can be diffused, added to a steam inhalation, or applied (diluted) to the chest for instant relief.

- **Peppermint Oil**: Peppermint oil contains menthol, which provides a cooling sensation that helps open airways and improve breathing. It's particularly effective for treating nasal congestion, sinusitis, and colds. Peppermint oil can be diffused or applied topically (diluted) to the chest to reduce congestion and promote easier breathing.

- **Tea Tree Oil**: Tea tree oil is a powerful antimicrobial agent, making it effective in treating respiratory infections. It helps to fight bacteria and viruses that cause respiratory conditions like bronchitis, sinusitis, and colds. Diffusing tea tree oil or adding it to a steam inhalation can purify the air and relieve respiratory symptoms.

- **Thyme Oil**: Thyme oil is known for its ability to support the respiratory system, helping to treat coughs, colds, and bronchitis. It has strong antimicrobial properties that fight off infections and reduce inflammation in the respiratory tract. Thyme oil can be diffused or diluted and applied to the chest to improve lung function and reduce respiratory symptoms.

- **Ravensara Oil**: Ravensara oil is lesser-known but highly effective for respiratory issues. It is antiviral and decongestant, making it ideal for treating colds, flu, and other respiratory infections. Diffusing ravensara oil or using it in a steam inhalation can help open airways and relieve congestion.

Pain Relief and Muscle Recovery

Essential oils offer a natural, non-invasive way to manage pain and aid in muscle recovery. Whether you're dealing with chronic pain, sore muscles, or tension headaches, essential oils can provide relief by reducing inflammation, improving circulation, and soothing muscles.

- **Peppermint Oil**: The cooling and anti-inflammatory properties of peppermint oil make it highly effective for relieving muscle pain and tension. Its menthol content provides a soothing, cooling sensation that can reduce soreness and inflammation. Peppermint oil can be diluted with a carrier oil and massaged into sore muscles or applied to the temples to relieve tension headaches.

- **Lavender Oil**: Lavender oil's calming properties extend beyond its ability to relax the mind—it's also effective for soothing muscle tension and reducing pain. Its anti-inflammatory properties help relieve soreness, while its calming effect aids in muscle recovery. Lavender oil can be used in a bath, massage, or topical application (diluted) for pain relief and relaxation.

- **Eucalyptus Oil**: Eucalyptus oil has analgesic and anti-inflammatory properties, making it effective for reducing pain and inflammation in muscles and joints. It helps to increase circulation, which aids in muscle recovery after exercise or injury. Eucalyptus oil can be diluted and massaged into sore muscles or added to a warm bath to relieve pain.

- **Ginger Oil**: Ginger oil is a powerful anti-inflammatory oil that helps reduce muscle and joint pain, especially in cases of arthritis or injury. Its warming properties improve circulation and promote healing. Ginger oil can be diluted and applied topically to the affected area for pain relief.

- **Helichrysum Oil**: Known for its potent healing properties, helichrysum oil is effective for reducing pain, inflammation, and swelling. It is particularly helpful for healing muscle injuries, bruises, and joint pain. Helichrysum oil can be diluted and applied to the skin to promote recovery and reduce pain.

Essential Oils for Mental and Emotional Well-being

Reducing Stress and Anxiety

Essential oils have been used for centuries to promote relaxation and reduce stress, making them a natural remedy for today's fast-paced lifestyle. When we inhale certain essential oils, their aromatic compounds interact with the brain's limbic system, which governs emotions, memories, and stress responses. The calming effects of essential oils can help lower cortisol levels, ease tension, and create a sense of peace.

- **Lavender Oil**: Lavender is the most well-known essential oil for stress relief, thanks to its ability to calm the nervous system and promote relaxation. Studies have shown that inhaling lavender can reduce anxiety, lower blood pressure, and slow heart rate, making it an ideal choice for those experiencing chronic stress. Whether diffused, added to a bath, or applied topically, lavender oil helps to ease both physical and emotional tension.

- **Bergamot Oil**: Bergamot has a refreshing citrus scent with floral undertones, making it both uplifting and calming. This unique combination helps reduce stress and anxiety while simultaneously boosting mood. Bergamot oil's ability to lower cortisol levels has been demonstrated in studies, making it effective for managing stress-related symptoms. It can be diffused in stressful environments or applied topically (diluted) to promote a sense of calm.

- **Ylang Ylang Oil**: Ylang ylang is another calming oil that helps reduce feelings of stress and anxiety. Its sweet, floral scent promotes relaxation, balances emotions, and reduces the feeling of being overwhelmed. Ylang ylang works by lowering blood pressure and heart rate, helping the body enter a more relaxed state. Diffusing ylang ylang or using it in a massage oil blend can create a soothing environment, ideal for stress reduction.

- **Frankincense Oil**: Frankincense is known for its grounding and centering properties. It has been used for centuries in spiritual and religious practices to promote inner peace. Frankincense works by calming the mind, slowing down breathing, and reducing stress-induced tension. Whether used in meditation or added to a diffuser, frankincense helps create a tranquil atmosphere, easing stress and promoting relaxation.

- **Clary Sage Oil**: Clary sage is particularly effective for relieving stress and anxiety related to hormonal imbalances. It has calming and uplifting effects, helping to reduce feelings of tension and emotional overwhelm. When inhaled or applied topically (diluted), clary sage can promote mental clarity and emotional balance, making it useful for managing stress and anxiety.

Managing Depression and Emotional Balance

Essential oils can be a powerful tool in managing symptoms of depression and promoting emotional balance. Their mood-enhancing properties come from their ability to stimulate the release of neurotransmitters like serotonin and dopamine, which are associated with feelings of happiness and well-being. While essential oils aren't a cure for depression, they can be part of a holistic approach to emotional health.

- **Rose Oil**: Rose essential oil is widely regarded as one of the most effective oils for lifting the mood and managing depression. Its rich, floral aroma has been shown to increase feelings of self-worth, reduce anxiety, and improve emotional well-being. Rose oil can be diffused or applied (diluted) to the skin to help ease feelings of sadness and promote emotional healing.

- **Jasmine Oil**: Jasmine oil is known for its uplifting and energizing properties, making it effective for managing symptoms of depression. Its sweet, floral scent stimulates the release of serotonin, promoting feelings of optimism and joy. Jasmine oil can be diffused to create a positive atmosphere or applied topically (with a carrier oil) to boost mood and emotional balance.

- **Chamomile Oil**: Chamomile is soothing and calming, often used to alleviate feelings of sadness and depression. Its gentle, floral aroma helps ease emotional tension and promote relaxation, making it especially useful for individuals experiencing anxiety or depressive symptoms. Chamomile oil can be diffused or used in a bath to calm the mind and promote emotional balance.

- **Sandalwood Oil**: Sandalwood has grounding properties that help to balance emotions and promote a sense of peace and stability. It's often used in meditation and spiritual practices to calm the mind and alleviate negative thoughts. Sandalwood oil can be diffused or applied topically to create a sense of emotional balance and well-being.

- **Clary Sage Oil**: Clary sage is also beneficial for managing depression, particularly in individuals who experience emotional imbalances related to hormonal fluctuations. Its uplifting and mood-enhancing properties can help ease feelings of sadness and promote a sense of optimism.

Enhancing Focus and Concentration

Essential oils can also help improve focus, mental clarity, and concentration. Certain oils have stimulating properties that increase blood flow to the brain, sharpen cognitive function, and enhance alertness. These oils are particularly useful for individuals who need to stay mentally sharp at work or during study sessions.

- **Rosemary Oil**: Rosemary is well-known for its ability to enhance memory, focus, and cognitive performance. Its stimulating properties increase blood circulation to the brain, which helps improve concentration and mental clarity. Studies have shown that inhaling rosemary oil can significantly boost memory retention and focus. Diffusing rosemary oil or applying it (diluted) to pulse points can enhance cognitive function during periods of intense mental work.

- **Peppermint Oil**: Peppermint is invigorating and refreshing, known to improve concentration and alertness. Its cooling properties help clear the mind, making it easier to focus on tasks and stay mentally sharp. Peppermint oil is often used to combat mental fatigue, boost energy, and enhance productivity. Diffusing peppermint oil or inhaling it directly can provide an instant mental boost, helping you stay focused and alert.

- **Lemon Oil**: Lemon oil's bright, refreshing scent stimulates the mind and enhances concentration. It is particularly useful for improving focus and mental clarity, especially during periods of stress or fatigue. Lemon oil can be diffused to create an energized and focused environment, or applied topically (diluted) to sharpen cognitive function.

- **Cedarwood Oil**: Cedarwood has grounding and balancing properties that help to calm the mind and improve focus. It is particularly effective for individuals who struggle with attention issues or mental fatigue. Cedarwood oil can be diffused to create a calm and focused atmosphere, or applied topically (diluted) to enhance concentration.

- **Basil Oil**: Basil oil is a powerful cognitive stimulant, helping to improve mental clarity and focus. Its refreshing and invigorating scent helps reduce mental fatigue, making it ideal for long periods of concentration. Basil oil can be diffused or applied to the temples (diluted) to enhance focus and cognitive performance.

Boosting Mood and Energy Levels

Essential oils can also serve as natural mood boosters and energy enhancers. When inhaled, certain oils stimulate the release of endorphins and serotonin, the body's natural "feel-good" chemicals. These oils are perfect for creating an uplifting atmosphere or for use during periods of low energy or motivation.

- **Grapefruit Oil**: Grapefruit essential oil is a bright and uplifting oil that helps to boost mood and energy levels. Its citrusy aroma stimulates the senses and promotes a positive, energized state of mind. Grapefruit oil can be diffused in the morning to start the day off on an energetic note or applied topically (diluted) to enhance mood and motivation.

- **Orange Oil**: Orange essential oil is known for its uplifting and mood-boosting properties. It helps reduce stress, combat fatigue, and promote feelings of happiness and positivity. Orange oil can be diffused or applied (diluted) to pulse points to increase energy levels and create an uplifting atmosphere.

- **Lemongrass Oil**: Lemongrass has a fresh, invigorating scent that helps to boost mood and energy levels. It is particularly effective for reducing mental fatigue and increasing alertness.

Lemongrass oil can be diffused to create a positive, energized environment or applied topically (diluted) for an instant mood lift.

- **Citrus Oils (Lemon, Lime, Bergamot)**: Citrus oils in general are great mood enhancers, thanks to their bright, fresh scents. These oils stimulate the senses and promote feelings of happiness and energy. Citrus oils can be blended and diffused throughout the day to keep energy levels high and mood positive.

- **Peppermint Oil**: In addition to its benefits for focus and concentration, peppermint oil is an excellent energy booster. Its refreshing scent helps to awaken the mind and body, making it ideal for use during periods of low energy or fatigue. Inhaling peppermint oil or applying it topically (diluted) can provide an instant energy boost and improve overall mood.

Essential Oils for Skin and Beauty Care

Acne Treatment and Skin Clarity

Essential oils offer a natural and effective way to treat acne and promote clear, healthy skin. Many essential oils contain antibacterial, anti-inflammatory, and balancing properties that can help reduce breakouts, soothe irritated skin, and prevent future blemishes. When used correctly, they can regulate sebum production, clear clogged pores, and reduce the appearance of acne scars.

- **Tea Tree Oil**: Tea tree oil is one of the most effective essential oils for treating acne. It has powerful antibacterial properties that help kill the acne-causing bacteria on the skin. Additionally, tea tree oil helps reduce inflammation, redness, and swelling associated with pimples. For spot treatment, dilute tea tree oil with a carrier oil (such as jojoba oil) and apply it directly to the affected area.

- **Lavender Oil**: Lavender oil is not only calming for the mind but also gentle on the skin. It helps to reduce inflammation and redness caused by acne, while also promoting the healing of acne scars. Lavender oil's antibacterial properties help prevent future breakouts, making it a great choice for people with sensitive or acne-prone skin.

- **Rosemary Oil**: Rosemary oil helps to reduce excess oil production, which can lead to clogged pores and breakouts. Its antimicrobial properties make it an effective choice for reducing the bacteria on the skin that causes acne. Rosemary oil can be diluted and applied to the face to prevent breakouts and promote clear skin.

- **Frankincense Oil**: Frankincense is a great option for treating acne, especially if scarring is a concern. Its healing properties help reduce the appearance of scars while promoting cell regeneration. Frankincense oil also helps balance the skin's oil production, preventing further breakouts while calming the skin.

- **Geranium Oil**: Geranium oil is another fantastic oil for balancing sebum production. It helps to reduce acne breakouts by controlling oil production and tightening pores. Geranium oil is also effective at reducing the appearance of acne scars and promoting a more even complexion.

Anti-Aging Properties of Essential Oils

As we age, the skin's ability to repair itself and produce collagen decreases, leading to wrinkles, fine lines, and loss of elasticity. Essential oils can be a powerful ally in fighting these signs of aging, thanks to their antioxidant, cell-regenerating, and collagen-boosting properties. Many essential oils also help hydrate and firm the skin, giving it a youthful, radiant glow.

- **Frankincense Oil**: Known for its anti-aging benefits, frankincense oil promotes the regeneration of healthy cells and reduces the appearance of wrinkles and fine lines. It also helps tighten and tone the skin, improving elasticity. Frankincense oil is a popular ingredient in many anti-aging serums due to its ability to reduce dark spots and improve skin texture.

- **Rosehip Oil**: Rosehip oil is packed with vitamins A and C, which are essential for skin renewal and collagen production. It helps reduce the appearance of fine lines, wrinkles, and age spots while promoting an even skin tone. Rosehip oil is deeply hydrating, making it perfect for mature skin that needs extra moisture.

- **Sandalwood Oil**: Sandalwood oil is prized for its soothing and anti-inflammatory properties, making it effective for reducing the appearance of fine lines and wrinkles. It helps improve skin texture and tone while keeping the skin hydrated. Sandalwood oil is often used in anti-aging formulations to promote smooth, youthful skin.

- **Myrrh Oil**: Myrrh oil is rich in antioxidants, which protect the skin from damage caused by free radicals. It also promotes skin regeneration, helping to reduce the appearance of fine lines and sagging skin. Myrrh oil can be blended with other essential oils to create a powerful anti-aging treatment.

- **Ylang Ylang Oil**: Ylang ylang is known for its ability to promote skin elasticity and combat the signs of aging. Its regenerative properties help reduce the appearance of fine lines and wrinkles, while its hydrating properties improve skin texture and softness. Ylang ylang oil is often used in anti-aging creams and serums.

Hair Care: Promoting Growth and Scalp Health

Essential oils can be highly beneficial for promoting hair growth, improving scalp health, and addressing common hair issues such as dandruff, dryness, and thinning. These oils nourish the scalp, improve blood circulation, and strengthen hair follicles, resulting in healthier, thicker hair.

- **Rosemary Oil**: Rosemary oil is widely known for its ability to stimulate hair growth and improve scalp health. It increases blood circulation to the scalp, which helps promote the growth of new hair. Rosemary oil can also prevent hair thinning and reduce dandruff. To use rosemary oil for hair growth, dilute it with a carrier oil and massage it into your scalp regularly.

- **Peppermint Oil**: Peppermint oil is invigorating and helps stimulate blood flow to the scalp, which encourages hair growth. It also has antimicrobial properties that help maintain a healthy scalp and reduce dandruff. The cooling sensation of peppermint oil can soothe an itchy scalp and promote healthy hair growth. Dilute peppermint oil and apply it to the scalp for best results.

- **Lavender Oil**: Lavender oil helps improve scalp health by promoting circulation and reducing stress, which can contribute to hair loss. It also has antimicrobial properties that help prevent scalp infections and dandruff. Lavender oil can be used to moisturize the scalp, strengthen hair follicles, and promote hair growth.

- **Cedarwood Oil**: Cedarwood oil is effective in promoting hair growth by stimulating the hair follicles and increasing circulation to the scalp. It also helps balance the production of oil on the scalp, preventing dryness or excess oiliness. Cedarwood oil is often used in hair care formulations to reduce hair loss and improve scalp health.

- **Tea Tree Oil**: Tea tree oil is a powerful antibacterial and antifungal agent that helps maintain a healthy scalp. It's particularly effective for treating dandruff and soothing an itchy scalp. Tea tree oil helps unblock hair follicles, promoting healthy hair growth. To use tea tree oil, dilute it with a carrier oil and massage it into your scalp to treat dandruff and encourage hair growth.

DIY Essential Oil Beauty Recipes

Creating your own DIY beauty products using essential oils is not only fun but also allows you to customize the products to suit your skin and hair care needs. Here are a few easy-to-make beauty recipes that harness the power of essential oils for radiant skin and healthy hair.

- **Tea Tree and Lavender Acne Spot Treatment**:
  - Ingredients:
    - 2 drops Tea Tree Oil
    - 2 drops Lavender Oil
    - 1 teaspoon Jojoba Oil (or another carrier oil)
  - Instructions: Mix the oils together and apply a small amount to acne spots using a cotton swab. Leave it on overnight to reduce inflammation and heal blemishes.
- **Anti-Aging Face Serum**:
  - Ingredients:
    - 5 drops Frankincense Oil
    - 5 drops Rosehip Oil
    - 3 drops Lavender Oil
    - 1 tablespoon Jojoba Oil (or another carrier oil)
  - Instructions: Combine all ingredients in a dark glass dropper bottle. Apply a few

drops to the face and neck after cleansing, focusing on areas with fine lines and wrinkles.

- **Rosemary Hair Growth Oil**:
  - Ingredients:
    - 5 drops Rosemary Oil
    - 3 drops Peppermint Oil
    - 2 drops Lavender Oil
    - 2 tablespoons Coconut Oil (or another carrier oil)
  - Instructions: Mix the oils in a small bottle. Massage the mixture into the scalp and let it sit for at least 30 minutes before washing it out. Use this treatment 1-2 times per week to promote hair growth.
- **Soothing Lavender and Chamomile Face Mask**:
  - Ingredients:
    - 2 tablespoons Kaolin Clay
    - 1 tablespoon Aloe Vera Gel
    - 3 drops Lavender Oil
    - 2 drops Chamomile Oil

- Water (as needed)
    - Instructions: Mix the clay, aloe vera, and essential oils together, adding water as needed to form a paste. Apply the mask to your face and leave it on for 10-15 minutes before rinsing off with warm water. This mask helps calm irritated skin and promote a clear complexion.

- **Coconut and Lavender Body Scrub**:
    - Ingredients:
        - 1/2 cup Coconut Oil
        - 1 cup Sugar
        - 5 drops Lavender Oil
        - 3 drops Frankincense Oil
    - Instructions: Combine all ingredients in a bowl and mix well. Use the scrub in the shower to exfoliate the skin, leaving it soft and hydrated.

Essential Oils for Home and Lifestyle

Creating a Toxin-Free Home with Essential Oils

In today's world, many household products contain harmful chemicals and toxins that can impact your health and the environment. Essential oils offer a natural alternative to conventional cleaning and home care products, allowing you to create a toxin-free living space. By incorporating essential oils into your cleaning routines, you can reduce exposure to harmful substances while still maintaining a clean, fresh-smelling home. Essential oils provide antimicrobial, antifungal, and antiviral benefits, making them ideal for cleaning and disinfecting surfaces, purifying the air, and promoting overall wellness.

- **Lemon Oil**: Lemon oil is a powerful natural cleaner, known for its antibacterial and antiviral properties. It's excellent for cutting through grease, grime, and stains, making it a versatile addition to any cleaning routine. Lemon oil also has a fresh, uplifting scent, which makes it perfect for freshening the air and deodorizing spaces.

- **Tea Tree Oil**: Tea tree oil is one of the most potent antimicrobial essential oils, capable of killing bacteria, viruses, and fungi. This makes it ideal for disinfecting surfaces in the kitchen, bathroom, and other high-touch areas in the home. Its strong antiseptic properties also make tea tree oil effective in cleaning mold and mildew.

- **Eucalyptus Oil**: Eucalyptus oil is known for its powerful antiviral and antibacterial properties, which can help eliminate germs and purify the air. It can be added to natural cleaning solutions to disinfect surfaces, or diffused to promote a clean and refreshing environment. Its fresh scent also helps eliminate odors, leaving your home smelling crisp and clean.

- **Lavender Oil**: Lavender oil not only has a calming scent but also offers mild antibacterial properties, making it a great choice for creating a toxin-free home. It's gentle enough to be used in laundry, linen sprays, or as a natural air freshener. Lavender oil can also help repel insects like moths from closets or linens.

Cleaning and Purifying with Essential Oils

Essential oils can be incorporated into homemade cleaning products to clean and purify your home effectively, without the use of harsh chemicals. Whether you're disinfecting kitchen counters, cleaning windows, or scrubbing floors, essential oils provide a natural and safe way to maintain a sparkling home.

- **All-Purpose Cleaner:**
  - Ingredients:
    - 1 cup white vinegar
    - 1 cup water
    - 10 drops Lemon Oil
    - 10 drops Tea Tree Oil
  - Instructions: Combine all ingredients in a spray bottle and shake well. Use this

all-purpose cleaner to disinfect countertops, sinks, bathroom surfaces, and more. The combination of lemon and tea tree oils offers a powerful antimicrobial punch, while vinegar helps to break down grease and grime.

- **Glass Cleaner**:
    - Ingredients:
        - 1/4 cup white vinegar
        - 1/4 cup rubbing alcohol
        - 1 tablespoon cornstarch
        - 10 drops Peppermint Oil
    - Instructions: Mix all ingredients in a spray bottle. Shake well before using. Spray on windows or mirrors and wipe clean with a microfiber cloth. Peppermint oil adds a refreshing scent and helps repel dust.
- **Wood Polish**:
    - Ingredients:
        - 1/4 cup olive oil
        - 1/4 cup white vinegar

- 10 drops Lemon Oil
        - 5 drops Cedarwood Oil
    - Instructions: Mix the ingredients in a small spray bottle. Shake well before use. Spray onto wooden surfaces and buff with a soft cloth. Lemon oil helps remove dirt, while cedarwood oil enhances the wood's natural shine and fragrance.

- **Air Purifying Blend**:
    - Ingredients:
        - 4 drops Eucalyptus Oil
        - 4 drops Lemon Oil
        - 3 drops Tea Tree Oil
        - 3 drops Peppermint Oil
    - Instructions: Add the oils to a diffuser and let it run for 15-30 minutes in your living areas. This blend helps purify the air, eliminate germs, and leave your home smelling fresh and clean.

Natural Insect Repellents and Home Fresheners

Many commercial insect repellents and air fresheners are loaded with synthetic fragrances and chemicals that can irritate the skin or respiratory system. Essential oils provide a natural, effective alternative for repelling insects and freshening your home. Their potent aromas and natural insecticidal properties make them a safe and eco-friendly choice for keeping pests at bay and maintaining a pleasant-smelling environment.

- **Citronella Oil**: Citronella oil is one of the most well-known natural insect repellents, particularly effective against mosquitoes. It can be diffused outdoors or applied topically (with dilution) to prevent bug bites. Citronella oil can also be added to homemade sprays for use around doors and windows to keep insects out of the home.

- **Lavender Oil**: In addition to its calming properties, lavender oil is a natural insect repellent. It helps keep mosquitoes, moths, flies, and other bugs away. Lavender can be used in sachets to protect clothing and linens from moths, or it can be mixed with water and sprayed around windows and doors as a gentle, non-toxic bug repellent.

- **Peppermint Oil**: Peppermint oil is highly effective at repelling ants, spiders, and rodents. Its strong scent overwhelms these pests, making it difficult for them to find food or nesting areas. To use peppermint oil as a natural insect repellent, mix 10 drops of peppermint oil with water in a spray bottle and spray around entry points like windows, doors, or cracks in the foundation.

- **Eucalyptus Oil**: Eucalyptus oil works well to repel ticks, fleas, and other insects. It can be mixed with water and sprayed in areas where pests are a problem, or it can be diffused to keep bugs at bay. Eucalyptus oil can also be applied to clothing or outdoor gear to repel ticks during hikes or outdoor activities.

- **DIY Air Freshener**:
  - Ingredients:
    - 1/2 cup distilled water
    - 1/4 cup rubbing alcohol
    - 10 drops Lavender Oil
    - 10 drops Lemon Oil
  - Instructions: Mix the ingredients in a spray bottle and shake well. Spray in the air or onto linens and upholstery to freshen your home. Lavender and lemon oils will eliminate odors while leaving a fresh, clean scent.

Essential Oils for Pets: Safety and Usage

While essential oils can provide many health benefits for humans, it's important to use them cautiously around pets. Some essential oils are safe for pets in diluted amounts, while others can be toxic. When used correctly, certain essential oils can help soothe anxiety, repel fleas and ticks, and improve your pet's overall well-being.

Always consult a veterinarian before introducing essential oils to your pets, especially if they have pre-existing health conditions.

- **Safe Essential Oils for Pets**:
  - **Lavender Oil**: Lavender oil is one of the safest essential oils to use around pets. It helps to reduce anxiety and promote calm in dogs and cats. Lavender can be diffused in small amounts or diluted and applied topically to help calm an anxious pet during stressful situations, such as thunderstorms or vet visits.
  - **Chamomile Oil**: Chamomile oil is soothing and gentle, helping to calm anxiety and promote restful sleep for pets. It can be diffused or used topically (properly diluted) to help with stress-related issues.
  - **Cedarwood Oil**: Cedarwood oil is effective at repelling fleas and ticks and is generally safe for pets when diluted. It

can be applied topically (diluted with a carrier oil) to your pet's bedding or collar to help keep pests away.

- ○ **Frankincense Oil**: Frankincense is safe for pets and can be used to promote a sense of calm. It can also support the immune system and reduce inflammation in pets.

- **Essential Oils to Avoid**: Some essential oils can be toxic to pets, even in small amounts. Oils such as **tea tree, eucalyptus, peppermint, citrus oils, pine**, and **wintergreen** should be avoided as they can cause respiratory distress, skin irritation, or toxicity if ingested.

- **How to Use Essential Oils Safely Around Pets**:
  - ○ **Diffusing**: When diffusing essential oils around pets, make sure the room is well-ventilated, and allow your pet to leave the room if they choose. Avoid placing diffusers directly near your pet's sleeping or eating areas.

- ○ **Topical Application**: If using essential oils topically on your pet, always dilute the oil with a carrier oil (such as coconut oil) and apply sparingly. Never apply oils directly to your pet's nose, ears, eyes, or paws.

- ○ **Insect Repellent Spray**: You can make a natural flea and tick repellent for your pets by combining 10 drops of lavender oil with 1 cup of water in a spray bottle. Lightly mist your pet's fur (avoiding the face) before walks or outdoor play to repel fleas and ticks.

Safety and Precautions

Potential Risks and Allergic Reactions

While essential oils offer many health and wellness benefits, it's important to recognize that they are highly concentrated plant extracts, and improper use can lead to adverse reactions. Some individuals may experience allergic reactions, skin irritation, or even toxicity if oils are not used with caution. Understanding the potential risks associated with essential oils can help ensure their safe and effective use.

- **Skin Irritation and Sensitization**: One of the most common risks associated with essential oils is skin irritation, which can occur when oils are applied directly to the skin without proper dilution. Sensitization refers to an allergic response that develops after repeated exposure to an essential oil, resulting in rashes, redness, or itching. To avoid these reactions, always dilute essential oils with a carrier oil (such as coconut or jojoba oil) before applying them to the skin. A patch test on a small area of skin, like the inner arm, is recommended to check for any allergic reactions.

- **Respiratory Issues**: Inhaling essential oils directly or diffusing them in large quantities can sometimes cause respiratory irritation, especially in individuals with asthma or other respiratory conditions. Strong oils like eucalyptus, tea tree, or peppermint may exacerbate breathing problems in sensitive individuals. It's important to use essential oils in well-ventilated areas and start with small amounts to ensure they are well tolerated.

- **Eye and Mucous Membrane Irritation**: Essential oils should never be applied directly to the eyes or mucous membranes (such as inside the nose or mouth) as they can cause severe irritation or even chemical burns. If essential oil accidentally gets into the eyes, rinse immediately with a carrier oil (not water) and seek medical advice if irritation persists.

- **Ingestion Risks**: Some essential oils are safe for internal use, but many are not and can be toxic if ingested. It's crucial to consult a healthcare professional before taking any essential oils internally. Ingesting oils like wintergreen, eucalyptus, or tea tree can lead to serious health complications, including poisoning.

Essential Oils to Avoid for Pregnant Women, Children, and Pets

Pregnant women, children, and pets are more vulnerable to the effects of essential oils, and certain oils should be avoided entirely to prevent adverse reactions. Always exercise caution when using essential oils in these populations, and consult a healthcare provider before use.

- **Pregnant Women**: During pregnancy, certain essential oils can stimulate uterine contractions or affect hormone levels, which may lead to complications. Pregnant women should avoid oils that are known to cause these effects, including:

- Clary Sage
- Rosemary
- Cinnamon
- Wintergreen
- Jasmine
- Aniseed
- Sage
- Fennel
- Thyme

- Oils like lavender, chamomile, and ylang-ylang are generally considered safe during pregnancy when properly diluted, but it's always best to consult with a healthcare provider before use.

- **Children**: Children have more sensitive skin and respiratory systems than adults, making them more susceptible to adverse reactions from essential oils. It's important to dilute oils more heavily when using them on children and avoid diffusing strong oils in enclosed spaces. Essential oils to avoid for children include:
  - Eucalyptus
  - Peppermint

- o   Wintergreen

- o   Birch

- o   Rosemary

- o   Sage

- o   Tea Tree (for children under 6)

- Safe options for children (when properly diluted) include lavender, chamomile, and frankincense. However, always do a patch test and avoid using oils on children's faces or hands, as they might accidentally ingest the oil.

- **Pets**: Some essential oils can be toxic to pets, especially cats and dogs. Cats, in particular, lack the liver enzymes necessary to process certain compounds found in essential oils, making them more vulnerable to toxicity. Essential oils to avoid around pets include:

  - o   Tea Tree

  - o   Eucalyptus

  - o   Citrus oils (orange, lemon, lime)

  - o   Peppermint

  - o   Pine

  - o   Cinnamon

- ○ Wintergreen
- Oils like lavender, chamomile, and cedarwood are generally safe for pets when used in small amounts and properly diluted. Avoid diffusing oils in spaces where your pets cannot leave, and never apply oils directly to their skin without veterinary guidance.

Understanding Phototoxicity and Sun Sensitivity

Phototoxicity occurs when certain essential oils increase the skin's sensitivity to sunlight, leading to sunburn, blistering, or skin discoloration when exposed to UV rays. This reaction is primarily associated with citrus oils, although other oils can also cause phototoxicity.

- **Phototoxic Oils**: The most common phototoxic essential oils are those derived from citrus fruits, as they contain compounds called furanocoumarins, which can cause sun sensitivity. Phototoxic oils include:
  - ○ Bergamot

- Lemon
    - Lime
    - Grapefruit
    - Bitter Orange

- **How to Avoid Phototoxic Reactions**: If you use any phototoxic oils topically, avoid direct sun exposure for at least 12-24 hours after application, depending on the oil and its concentration. To safely use citrus oils on the skin without risk of phototoxicity, you can either apply them in areas not exposed to sunlight or use steam-distilled versions of the oils, which do not contain furanocoumarins.

Proper Handling and Avoiding Overuse

Essential oils are potent substances, and using them correctly is key to avoiding adverse effects such as skin irritation, allergic reactions, or toxicity. Overuse or improper handling can lead to negative outcomes, so it's important to practice safe usage habits.

- **Dilution Is Key**: Essential oils should never be applied directly to the skin without dilution. A typical dilution ratio for topical use is 1-2% essential oil to carrier oil, which translates to 5-10 drops of essential oil per 1 ounce (30 mL) of carrier oil. For children, elderly individuals, or those with sensitive skin, an even lower dilution (0.5-1%) is recommended.

- **Rotate Oils**: To avoid sensitization, which can develop with repeated use of the same essential oil over time, rotate the oils you use and give your skin regular breaks from essential oil applications. Sensitization can lead to long-term allergic reactions, making it important to switch up your oils periodically.

- **Use Appropriate Amounts**: More is not better when it comes to essential oils. Using too many drops in a diffuser or applying undiluted oils to the skin can cause headaches, dizziness, or skin irritation. Stick to recommended doses, and if you're new to essential oils, start with small amounts to gauge your tolerance.

- **Proper Storage**: Store essential oils in dark, glass bottles in a cool, dry place away from sunlight. Heat and light can degrade the quality of the oils over time, reducing their effectiveness. Always ensure the cap is tightly sealed to prevent evaporation and contamination.

- **Avoid Ingestion**: Unless under the supervision of a qualified healthcare professional, avoid ingesting essential oils. Ingesting certain oils can lead to serious health complications, including toxicity or damage to internal organs. Essential oils are highly concentrated and can be harmful when consumed improperly.

- **Discontinue Use if Reactions Occur**: If you experience any adverse reactions (skin irritation, headaches, respiratory issues, etc.) while using essential oils, discontinue use immediately. Seek medical advice if the symptoms persist, and consider switching to a different oil that suits your body's needs better.

Making Essential Oils a Part of Your Daily Routine

Incorporating Essential Oils into Morning and Evening Rituals

Incorporating essential oils into your daily routines can transform both your mornings and evenings into rejuvenating rituals that promote overall wellness. Essential oils can help energize and focus your mind in the morning, while providing relaxation and calm at night. Creating consistent habits around these oils can improve your physical, emotional, and mental health.

Morning Rituals

The morning sets the tone for the day, and using essential oils in your routine can help boost energy levels, improve focus, and create a positive mindset.

- **Peppermint and Lemon for Energy**: Kickstart your day with invigorating oils like peppermint and lemon. Peppermint oil boosts energy levels and improves mental clarity, while lemon oil provides an uplifting, refreshing scent that promotes a sense of optimism. Simply add a few drops to a diffuser while getting ready, or dilute them with a carrier oil and apply to your pulse points.

- **Rosemary for Focus**: If you need to focus and stay mentally sharp throughout the day, rosemary oil is a great choice. Its stimulating properties can help improve memory and concentration. Try adding rosemary oil to your morning shower by placing a few drops on a washcloth and letting the steam release the oil's aroma. You can also diffuse it in your workspace to enhance productivity.

- **Orange for Uplifted Mood**: Orange oil is a natural mood booster. Its bright, citrusy aroma lifts the spirits and helps set a positive tone for the day. You can add a few drops of orange oil to your body lotion or blend it with peppermint in a diffuser to create a refreshing and joyful environment.

Evening Rituals

As the day winds down, essential oils can help transition your mind and body into a state of relaxation, preparing you for a restful night's sleep. Evening rituals with essential oils promote calm, relaxation, and emotional balance.

- **Lavender for Relaxation**: Lavender is one of the best essential oils for promoting relaxation and reducing stress. Incorporate it into your evening by diffusing lavender in your bedroom for 30 minutes before bed. You can also create a calming bath by adding a few drops to warm water, or apply diluted lavender oil to your temples, neck, or wrists to unwind.

- **Chamomile for Stress Relief**: Chamomile is another calming oil that helps ease anxiety and promotes deep relaxation. It's ideal for a calming tea blend or as part of your evening skincare routine. Add chamomile oil to a carrier oil and use it in a nighttime massage to help relieve tension and stress.

- **Frankincense for Sleep**: Frankincense helps calm the mind, slow down breathing, and prepare the body for sleep. Diffusing frankincense in your bedroom or adding a drop to your pillow can help you drift off into a deep, peaceful sleep. Its grounding effect also makes it a great addition to meditation or deep breathing exercises before bed.

Using Essential Oils in Meditation and Yoga Practice

Essential oils can enhance your meditation and yoga practice by promoting mental clarity, emotional grounding, and relaxation. Their ability to influence mood and create a calming atmosphere makes them perfect companions for mindfulness practices. When combined with deep breathing, essential oils can deepen your connection to your body and mind.

Meditation

- **Frankincense for Grounding**: Frankincense has been used for centuries in spiritual and religious practices due to its grounding and centering properties. It helps to calm the mind, deepen breathing, and promote a sense of peace. Diffuse frankincense during your meditation practice to create a tranquil space, or apply a drop to your palms, rub them together, and inhale deeply before beginning your practice.

- **Sandalwood for Spirituality**: Sandalwood is known for its ability to promote spiritual awareness and inner peace. Its rich, woody aroma can enhance your meditation practice by helping you stay present and grounded. Sandalwood oil can be used in a diffuser or applied (diluted) to the pulse points before meditating to encourage deep focus.

- **Clary Sage for Emotional Release**: Clary sage is ideal for meditation when you're seeking emotional balance and release. Its soothing properties help reduce anxiety and emotional tension, allowing you to let go of stress. Diffuse clary sage or apply a diluted drop to the soles of your feet to foster relaxation and openness during your practice.

Yoga

- **Peppermint for Invigoration**: Peppermint oil is perfect for energizing and invigorating your yoga practice. It opens the airways, improves circulation, and enhances focus, making it great for more active or flow-based yoga sessions. Add a few drops to your diffuser during practice or dilute and apply to your wrists before starting your yoga routine.

- **Lavender for Relaxation**: For more restorative or yin yoga practices, lavender oil is an excellent choice. It helps release muscle tension and promotes deep relaxation, allowing you to sink into poses and relax fully. You can diffuse lavender oil in your yoga space or apply it to your temples and neck before your practice.

- **Eucalyptus for Breath Support**: Eucalyptus oil is great for opening up the respiratory system, making it easier to breathe deeply during yoga. Its fresh, clean scent promotes mental clarity and focus, making it ideal for Pranayama (breath work) or deep breathing exercises. Eucalyptus can be diffused or applied (diluted) to the chest and neck before your yoga session to enhance breath control.

Travel-Friendly Essential Oils for On-the-Go Health Support

Travel can often be stressful, but bringing along travel-friendly essential oils can help keep you grounded, healthy, and relaxed no matter where you are. Essential oils are perfect for relieving travel-related discomforts like jet lag, headaches, stress, and digestive issues.

- **Peppermint for Headaches and Nausea**: Peppermint oil is a must-have travel companion due to its ability to relieve headaches, nausea, and motion sickness. Apply a diluted drop to your temples or wrists when you feel queasy, or inhale directly from the bottle for quick relief. Peppermint can also help alleviate fatigue and mental fog during long flights or road trips.

- **Lavender for Stress and Sleep**: Lavender oil is ideal for promoting calm and relaxation while traveling. It can be used to reduce anxiety, promote restful sleep, and ease travel-related stress. Carry a small roller bottle of diluted lavender oil to apply to your pulse points when feeling overwhelmed, or add a drop to your travel pillow for better sleep on the go.

- **Tea Tree Oil for Immune Support**: Travel exposes you to new environments and potential germs, making tea tree oil a great addition to your travel kit. Its antimicrobial properties help protect against bacteria and viruses. You can apply tea tree oil (diluted) to cuts or scrapes, or diffuse it in your hotel room to purify the air.

- **Lemon Oil for Energy and Detoxification**: Lemon oil helps boost energy levels, improve mood, and aid in detoxification, making it a great oil to carry while traveling. A drop of lemon oil added to your water (if food-grade) can help support digestion and detoxify the body, while diffusing it in a travel diffuser can keep you feeling fresh and energized.

- **Eucalyptus for Respiratory Health**: Eucalyptus oil can help open airways and ease congestion, especially when traveling to different climates or environments. It's great for keeping your respiratory system healthy and clear. A few drops of eucalyptus in a portable diffuser or inhaled from a tissue can support clear breathing during your journey.

Long-Term Benefits of Integrating Essential Oils into Everyday Life

Integrating essential oils into your daily routine has long-term benefits for your physical, mental, and emotional health. By consistently using essential oils, you can create rituals that support your well-being, reduce stress, and improve overall quality of life.

- **Stress Management**: Over time, regular use of essential oils like lavender, frankincense, and chamomile can help reduce chronic stress and anxiety. Establishing routines with these oils, such as diffusing them during meditation or applying them before bed, can help your body and mind enter a more relaxed, balanced state.

- **Improved Sleep**: Essential oils like lavender, sandalwood, and cedarwood can promote better sleep habits. Long-term use can help regulate your sleep cycle, allowing you to fall asleep more easily and wake up feeling refreshed. Over time, this can lead to improved mood, cognitive function, and overall energy levels.

- **Boosted Immunity**: Regular use of immune-supporting oils like tea tree, eucalyptus, and lemon can strengthen your body's natural defenses against illness. Diffusing these oils regularly or incorporating them into your cleaning routine can help reduce the spread of germs and bacteria in your home, keeping you and your family healthier in the long run.

- **Enhanced Emotional Balance**: Essential oils like rose, jasmine, and ylang-ylang are powerful tools for balancing emotions and improving mood. When used consistently, they can help reduce feelings of depression, anxiety, and emotional imbalance. Over time, you'll notice more emotional stability and resilience in stressful situations.

- **Physical Wellness**: Essential oils with anti-inflammatory and pain-relieving properties, such as peppermint, eucalyptus, and ginger, can help alleviate chronic pain, muscle tension, and headaches. Regular use can lead to improved physical health and reduced reliance on over-the-counter pain medications.

By incorporating essential oils into your everyday life, you can enjoy lasting benefits for your body, mind, and home. The key is to develop consistent routines that work for your lifestyle and wellness goals.

Conclusion

As we come to the end of this journey into the world of essential oils, it's important to reflect on the natural healing powers that have been used for centuries to promote health and wellness. From ancient civilizations to modern-day wellness practices, essential oils have stood the test of time as a natural, effective way to support physical, mental, and emotional well-being. The knowledge you've gained throughout this book is just the beginning of what essential oils can offer in your journey toward natural healing.

By learning how to incorporate these powerful oils into your daily routines—whether it's through morning rituals to boost energy, evening routines to promote relaxation, or using oils to treat specific health concerns—you're stepping into a world where nature's most potent tools are at your disposal. Essential oils are not just about quick fixes; they offer a holistic approach to well-being that can have a profound impact on your life.

The beauty of essential oils is in their versatility. Whether you're looking to relieve stress, boost your immune system, clear your skin, or support a healthy home, there's an essential oil (or blend) to meet your needs. With a little experimentation, patience, and awareness, you can unlock the full potential of these natural remedies.

Throughout this exploration of essential oils, we've covered everything from their ancient origins and extraction methods to their wide-ranging therapeutic properties. We've discussed how to integrate them into various aspects of your life, from beauty and skincare to mental clarity and emotional balance.

The journey toward natural healing is a deeply personal one. It's about rediscovering the power of nature and making choices that align with your body's needs. Essential oils allow you to return to a more natural state of health, relying on the earth's resources rather than synthetic products or harsh chemicals. This journey is not about perfection or following rigid protocols—it's about listening to your body and using the tools nature has provided to enhance your well-being.

Continuing on this path, remember that healing is a lifelong process. Essential oils can be a powerful support system, but they work best when integrated into a balanced lifestyle that includes good nutrition, exercise, mindfulness, and self-care.

As you close this book, I encourage you to take charge of your health and well-being by incorporating essential oils into your everyday life. Essential oils are more than just a luxury or an occasional indulgence—they are a practical, accessible way to take control of your physical, emotional, and mental health. The knowledge you now possess empowers you to make informed choices about your well-being, and these natural remedies can be integrated into a balanced, holistic lifestyle.

Start small by incorporating a few essential oils into your daily routine. Diffuse lavender to unwind after a long day, use tea tree oil in your skincare routine, or try peppermint oil to boost focus during work. As you grow more comfortable with these oils, you'll find yourself reaching for them as your go-to solution for everything from stress relief to home cleaning.

Taking control of your health means embracing the idea that natural remedies, like essential oils, can support your body's innate ability to heal and thrive. You don't need to rely solely on synthetic medications or chemical-laden products when you have access to the healing properties of nature right at your fingertips.

Remember, essential oils are just one piece of the puzzle. They work best when combined with a healthy diet, regular exercise, stress management techniques, and other wellness practices. The more you integrate them into your life, the more you'll experience their transformative power.

Thank you for taking this journey into the world of essential oils. I hope this book has inspired you to embrace natural healing and make essential oils a meaningful part of your wellness routine. May these oils bring balance, health, and joy into your life for years to come.